Ke  Beginners

Preparing for Kegel Exercises

By

Darian Clayton
Copyright@2023

Table of Contents

CHAPTER 1 5

Introduction 5

  1.1 What Are Kegel Exercises?......5

  1.2 Benefits of Kegel Exercises 6

CHAPTER 2 11

Understanding Your Pelvic Floor....11

  2.1 Anatomy of the Pelvic Floor ..11

  2.2 Function of the Pelvic Floor Muscles..14

CHAPTER 3 18

Getting Started..................................18

  3.1 Preparing for Kegel Exercises 18

  3.2 Finding the Right Muscles 20

  3.3 Common Mistakes to Avoid ..22

CHAPTER 4 25

Basic Kegel Exercises 25

  4.1 Step-by-Step Instructions 25

4.2 How Many Repetitions and Sets? 30

4.3 When and Where to Do Kegel Exercises..34

CHAPTER 5 40

Progressing Your Kegel Routine.....40

5.1 Intermediate Kegel Exercises.40

5.2 Advanced Kegel Exercises.....45

5.3 Tracking Your Progress 50

CHAPTER 6 56

Common Questions and Concerns ..56

6.1 Can You Overdo Kegel Exercises?......................................56

6.2 Troubleshooting Common Issues 61

6.3 Seeking Professional Guidance 67

CHAPTER 7 73

Incorporating Kegels into Daily Life 73

7.1 Kegels for Men 73

7.2 Kegels for Women 78

7.3 Maintaining a Healthy Pelvic Floor 83

CHAPTER 1

Introduction

1.1 What Are Kegel Exercises?

Kegel exercises, named after Dr. Arnold Kegel who introduced them in the 1940s, are a set of simple, yet highly effective, pelvic floor exercises designed to strengthen the muscles responsible for supporting the pelvic organs. These exercises primarily target the pelvic floor muscles, which consist of a group of muscles located at the base of the pelvis. The pelvic floor muscles play a vital role in various bodily functions, such as bladder and bowel control, sexual function, and providing support to the uterus and other pelvic organs in women.

Kegel exercises involve a series of voluntary contractions and relaxations of the pelvic floor muscles. The main muscle involved is the pubococcygeus muscle, which runs from the pubic bone to the tailbone. These exercises are accessible and can be done discreetly without the need for any special equipment, making them an ideal form of physical therapy for a variety of conditions and individuals of all genders.

1.2 Benefits of Kegel Exercises

The benefits of incorporating Kegel exercises into your routine are multifaceted and can positively impact several aspects of your physical and emotional well-being. Here are some of the key advantages:

1. Improved Pelvic Health: One of the primary benefits of Kegel exercises is the enhancement of pelvic health. Strengthening the pelvic floor muscles can help prevent or alleviate issues like urinary incontinence, fecal incontinence, and pelvic organ prolapse. These exercises are particularly beneficial for individuals who have given birth, as pregnancy and childbirth can weaken the pelvic floor muscles.

2. Urinary Incontinence Management: Kegel exercises are often recommended as a non-invasive treatment for urinary incontinence, a condition characterized by the involuntary leakage of urine. Strengthening the pelvic floor can help individuals regain control over their bladder, reducing the frequency and severity of leaks.

3. Enhanced Sexual Function: A strong pelvic floor is crucial for sexual health. Kegel exercises can lead to increased sexual satisfaction for both men and women. In women, these exercises can improve vaginal tightness and the ability to achieve orgasm, while in men, they can aid in controlling ejaculation and maintaining erections.

4. Preparation for Pregnancy and Postpartum Recovery: Women who practice Kegel exercises during pregnancy can experience an easier labor and delivery. These exercises can also help with postpartum recovery by restoring the strength and tone of the pelvic floor muscles.

5. Prostate Health: In men, Kegel exercises can support prostate health. These exercises can help improve urinary control, potentially reducing the risk of benign prostatic hyperplasia (BPH) and other prostate-related issues.

6. Increased Awareness and Mind-Body Connection: Engaging in Kegel exercises fosters a heightened awareness of the pelvic region and can establish a stronger connection between the mind and body. This increased awareness can have positive effects on overall bodily coordination and well-being.

7. Enhanced Quality of Life: Ultimately, the benefits of Kegel exercises extend to an improved overall quality of life. They empower individuals to take control of their pelvic health and enjoy greater confidence and comfort in everyday activities.

It's important to note that while Kegel exercises offer numerous advantages, they are not a one-size-fits-all solution. It's advisable to consult with a healthcare professional, such as a physical therapist, gynecologist, or urologist, to ensure that you are performing these exercises correctly and that they are suitable for your specific needs and health goals.

CHAPTER 2

Understanding Your Pelvic Floor

2.1 Anatomy of the Pelvic Floor

To fully comprehend the importance of Kegel exercises and their impact on pelvic health, it's essential to have a basic understanding of the anatomy of the pelvic floor. The pelvic floor is a group of muscles, ligaments, and connective tissues that form a hammock-like structure at the base of the pelvis. This complex network of tissues serves several critical functions, which include:

- **Levator Ani Muscles:** The pelvic floor is primarily composed of the levator ani muscles, which can be further divided into the pubococcygeus, iliococcygeus, and puborectalis muscles. These muscles extend from the pubic bone in the front to the coccyx (tailbone) at the back and laterally to the pelvic sidewalls. They are responsible for supporting the pelvic organs, such as the bladder, uterus (in women), and rectum.

- **Urogenital Diaphragm:** The urogenital diaphragm is a layer of connective tissue and muscle that forms the base of the pelvis. It supports the urethra and vagina in women and the urethra in men.

- **Perineum:** The perineum is the area between the genitals and the anus. It is a critical part of the pelvic floor and plays a role in sexual function and bowel control.

- **Sphincters:** The pelvic floor also contains sphincters, which are circular muscles that encircle the urethra and anus. These sphincters control the release of urine and feces.

- **Connective Tissues:** Ligaments and connective tissues provide structural support to the pelvic floor, helping to maintain the position of pelvic organs.

2.2 Function of the Pelvic Floor Muscles

Understanding the function of the pelvic floor muscles is crucial for appreciating why they matter in the context of Kegel exercises:

- **Support:** The primary function of the pelvic floor muscles is to provide support for the pelvic organs. They act like a sling, keeping the bladder, uterus (in women), and rectum in their proper positions. Weakened pelvic floor muscles can lead to pelvic organ prolapse, a condition where these organs descend from their normal positions.

- **Continence:** The pelvic floor muscles play a pivotal role in urinary and fecal continence.

They work in tandem with the sphincters to maintain control over the release of urine and stool. Strengthening these muscles can significantly improve one's ability to hold and release bodily waste voluntarily.

- **Sexual Function:** The pelvic floor is intimately linked to sexual function. In women, well-toned pelvic floor muscles contribute to vaginal tightness and can enhance sexual pleasure. In men, they aid in erectile function and control over ejaculation.

- **Core Stability:** These muscles are part of the body's core and contribute to overall stability. A strong core helps with balance, posture, and the prevention of lower back pain.

- **Childbirth:** During childbirth, the pelvic floor muscles stretch and accommodate the baby's passage through the birth canal. Strengthening these muscles before and after childbirth can aid in a smoother labor and faster postpartum recovery.

- **Bowel Function:** Pelvic floor muscles also influence bowel function by aiding in the control of bowel movements. Weak pelvic floor muscles can lead to issues like fecal incontinence.

The pelvic floor muscles are indispensable for various bodily functions, including support of pelvic organs, continence, sexual function, and core stability. By understanding the anatomy and function of these muscles, individuals can appreciate the significance of Kegel exercises in maintaining or improving pelvic health.

CHAPTER 3

Getting Started

3.1 Preparing for Kegel Exercises

Before embarking on your Kegel exercise journey, it's essential to make some preparations to ensure a smooth and effective experience:

- **Consult a Healthcare Professional:** If you have any underlying medical conditions, such as pelvic pain, incontinence, or recent pelvic surgery, it's advisable to consult a healthcare professional, such as a urologist, gynecologist, or physical therapist. They can provide guidance tailored to your specific needs and advise on the suitability of Kegel exercises.

- **Create a Routine:** Establish a consistent routine for your Kegel exercises. Determine when and where you will do them, and stick to this schedule. Consistency is key to experiencing the benefits of these exercises.

- **Comfortable Clothing:** Wear comfortable clothing that allows you to move freely during your exercises. You should feel at ease and relaxed while performing Kegels.

- **Privacy:** Kegel exercises are discreet and can be done anywhere, but you may prefer privacy as you get acquainted with them. Find a quiet, private space where you can focus on your exercises without distractions.

- **Empty Bladder:** Before starting your exercises, it's generally a good idea to empty your bladder. This reduces the risk of discomfort or interruptions during the exercises.

3.2 Finding the Right Muscles

Locating and engaging the correct muscles is a crucial step in Kegel exercises. Follow these steps to find the right muscles:

- **Stop the Flow:** One way to identify your pelvic floor

muscles is to interrupt the flow of urine while you're urinating. However, do not make a habit of this, as repeatedly stopping the flow of urine can lead to bladder issues.

- **Tightening Technique:** Another method is to visualize the muscles that you would use to prevent gas from passing or to stop the flow of urine. The muscles that contract in these situations are your pelvic floor muscles.

- **Finger Test:** If you're having trouble identifying these muscles, you can insert a clean finger into your vagina (for women) or rectum (for men). When you contract the right muscles, you should feel a gentle squeeze around your finger. This can help you ensure you're targeting the correct area.

3.3 Common Mistakes to Avoid

Avoiding common mistakes can enhance the effectiveness and safety of your Kegel exercises:

- **Overexertion:** One common mistake is overexerting the pelvic floor muscles. Do not forcefully contract these muscles; it's about control, not strength. Overexertion can lead to muscle fatigue and discomfort.

- **Holding Your Breath:** Remember to breathe regularly while doing Kegel exercises.

Holding your breath can lead to increased pressure in the pelvic area and may not yield the desired results.

- **Inconsistency:** To see progress, you must be consistent with your exercises. Skipping sessions or not following a routine can slow your progress.

- **Incorrect Muscles:** Ensure you are targeting the correct muscles. Some individuals inadvertently contract other muscles, such as the buttocks or abdomen, instead of the pelvic floor muscles. Focusing on the wrong muscles won't yield the desired results.

- **Improper Technique:** Proper form is crucial. Make sure you fully contract and then relax the pelvic floor muscles. Rushing through the exercises or not fully engaging and releasing these muscles can diminish their effectiveness.

By preparing adequately, finding the right muscles, and avoiding common mistakes, you can lay a solid foundation for your Kegel exercises and maximize their benefits for your pelvic health and overall well-being.

CHAPTER 4

Basic Kegel Exercises

4.1 Step-by-Step Instructions

Performing Kegel exercises correctly is essential to experience their full benefits. Here's a step-by-step guide on how to do basic Kegel exercises:

Step 1: Preparation

- Find a quiet, comfortable place where you can focus on your exercises without distractions.

- Sit, stand, or lie down in a relaxed position. You can

choose the position that is most comfortable for you.

Step 2: Identify Your Pelvic Floor Muscles

- Start by identifying your pelvic floor muscles. You can do this by using one of the following techniques:

    - Imagine stopping the flow of urine midstream. The muscles you engage to do this are your pelvic floor muscles.

    - Visualize the muscles you use to prevent passing gas. These are the same muscles.

    - For women, you can insert a clean finger into your vagina, and for men, into the rectum. When you contract the right muscles, you should feel a gentle squeeze around your finger.

Step 3: Perform the Exercise

- Take a deep breath in, and as you exhale, gently contract your pelvic floor muscles. It's essential to focus on the correct muscles and avoid using your abdomen, buttocks, or thighs.

Step 4: Hold and Release

- Hold the contraction for 3 to 5 seconds initially. As you progress, aim to hold for up to 10 seconds.

- After holding, release the muscles completely, allowing

them to relax for an equal duration (3 to 10 seconds).

Step 5: Repetitions and Sets

- Start with 10 repetitions for each session. Over time, gradually increase the number of repetitions until you reach a comfortable level.

- Aim to complete 3 sets of exercises per day.

Step 6: Consistency

- Consistency is key to seeing results. Make Kegel exercises a regular part of your routine.

Tips:

- Do not rush through the exercises. Focus on the quality of each contraction and relaxation.

- Breathe naturally throughout the exercise, and do not hold your breath.

- Avoid overexertion. These exercises are about control, not strength.

- Do not contract other muscles, such as your abdomen or buttocks, while performing Kegels.

- Stay patient. It may take a few weeks to notice significant improvements in pelvic health.

Kegel exercises are highly individual, and it's essential to adapt them to your comfort level. As you gain strength and control, you can increase the duration of contractions and the number of repetitions. For personalized guidance and to ensure you're performing Kegel exercises correctly, consider consulting a healthcare professional or physical therapist.

4.2 How Many Repetitions and Sets?

The number of repetitions and sets for Kegel exercises can vary depending on your individual needs, goals, and the advice of your healthcare professional. However, as a general guideline, here's an outline for how many repetitions and sets you can consider, especially if you're new to Kegel exercises:

Repetitions:

1. **Initial Phase:** Start with 10 repetitions for each session. This is a reasonable starting point for beginners and allows

you to become familiar with the exercises.

2. **Progression:** As you become more comfortable with the exercises and gain better control over your pelvic floor muscles, aim to gradually increase the number of repetitions. You can work your way up to 20-30 repetitions for each session.

Sets:

1. **Initial Phase:** Begin with one set of 10 repetitions per day. This serves as a foundation for your Kegel exercise routine.

2. **Progression:** Over time, work toward completing three sets of Kegel exercises per day. This means you will perform 10-30 repetitions in each of these sets.

Three sets are a commonly recommended goal for a well-rounded Kegel exercise routine.

Progress and Personalization:

- It's essential to listen to your body and adapt the number of repetitions and sets based on your comfort level and progress. Some individuals may progress more quickly than others.

- Remember that the effectiveness of Kegel exercises is not solely determined by the quantity of repetitions but also by the quality of the contractions and relaxations. Focus on engaging and releasing the pelvic floor muscles correctly.

- As you gain strength and control, you can also consider experimenting with different durations for both the contraction and relaxation phases. For instance, you may increase the contraction time to 10 seconds and maintain a 10-second relaxation period, but this should be done gradually and comfortably.

- If you experience any discomfort or pain during your exercises, or if you have specific pelvic health issues, it's highly recommended to consult a healthcare professional or physical therapist who can provide personalized guidance and help determine the appropriate number of repetitions and sets for your situation.

Ultimately, the key to successful Kegel exercises lies in maintaining consistency, gradual progression, and staying in tune with your body's responses. Tailoring your Kegel routine to your specific needs and goals will help you make the most of these exercises in promoting pelvic health and overall well-being.

4.3 When and Where to Do Kegel Exercises

Kegel exercises can be done discreetly in various settings and at different times to fit your schedule and preferences. Here's a guide on when and where to perform Kegel exercises:

When to Do Kegel Exercises:

1. **Morning Routine:** Some people find it beneficial to include Kegel exercises as part of their morning routine. This can help kickstart your day with a focus on pelvic health.

2. **During Daily Activities:** You can integrate Kegel exercises into your daily activities, such as when you're sitting at your desk, watching TV, or waiting in line. This discreet approach allows you to perform Kegels without drawing attention.

3. **Before or After Meals:** Incorporating Kegel exercises before or after meals is a convenient way to remember your routine. For example, you can do them while waiting for

your food to cook or during a post-dinner relaxation period.

4. **In Bed:** Some individuals prefer to do Kegel exercises before bedtime. This can help you unwind and establish a routine that supports your pelvic health.

5. **During Commutes:** If you have a daily commute, consider doing Kegel exercises while driving or on public transportation. Just be sure to maintain your focus on the road if you're the one driving.

6. **Scheduled Times:** You can set specific times during the day to perform your Kegel exercises. This might include once in the morning, once in the afternoon, and once before bedtime.

Where to Do Kegel Exercises:

1. **At Home:** You can comfortably do Kegel exercises at home in a private and relaxed environment. Find a quiet space where you won't be disturbed.

2. **Workplace:** If you have a private office or a secluded workspace, you can perform Kegel exercises during your workday without interruption. Alternatively, you can do them subtly at your desk without anyone noticing.

3. **Gym:** If you're comfortable, you can do Kegel exercises at the gym. However, it's advisable to do them in a less crowded area or during a quiet moment in your workout routine.

4. **Outdoors:** When you're in a park, on a walk, or in nature, you can also do Kegel exercises discreetly. Find a quiet spot to focus on your routine.

5. **Anywhere and Everywhere:** Kegel exercises are versatile and can be done virtually anywhere. The key is to focus on the correct muscles, maintain proper form, and be consistent with your routine.

The effectiveness of Kegel exercises depends on your consistency and the quality of your contractions and relaxations. It's essential to find a routine that works for you and to adapt your exercises to your daily life. Additionally, consult with a healthcare professional or physical therapist to ensure you're performing Kegel exercises correctly and that they are appropriate for your specific needs and goals.

CHAPTER 5

Progressing Your Kegel Routine

5.1 Intermediate Kegel Exercises

As you become more experienced with basic Kegel exercises and feel your pelvic floor muscles gaining strength, it's a good idea to progress to intermediate Kegel exercises. These exercises can further challenge and improve the endurance and coordination of your pelvic floor muscles. Here are some intermediate Kegel exercises to consider:

1. **Long Holds:** Instead of the typical 3- to 10-second holds in

basic Kegel exercises, try extending the duration of your contractions. Begin with 10-15 seconds and gradually increase the hold time as you become more proficient. Longer holds can enhance muscle endurance.

2. **Pulses:** After contracting your pelvic floor muscles, pulse or "flutter" them by repeatedly contracting and relaxing quickly for 10-15 seconds. This exercise can improve the rapid muscle response and coordination of your pelvic floor.

3. **Elevator Kegels:** Imagine your pelvic floor as an elevator with multiple levels. Start by contracting the muscles lightly (first floor) and gradually increase the intensity of the

contraction (second, third, and fourth floors), then release in the reverse order. This exercise encourages muscle control and coordination.

4. **Bridge Pose Kegels:** While doing a bridge pose (lying on your back with knees bent and feet flat on the floor, lifting your hips), contract your pelvic floor muscles and hold them while you maintain the bridge pose for 10-15 seconds. This exercise combines pelvic floor strengthening with core stability.

5. **Side-Lying Kegels:** Lie on your side with your knees bent and legs stacked. Contract your pelvic floor muscles while in this position, holding for 10-15 seconds. Side-lying Kegels help

target different areas of your pelvic floor.

6. **Advanced Quick Contractions:** In the advanced stage, practice quick and forceful contractions of your pelvic floor muscles, as if you're attempting to stop a sudden urge to urinate. Aim for 10-15 quick contractions in succession, then rest, and repeat for several sets.

7. **Use Props:** Introduce resistance or props, such as using a small exercise ball or resistance bands, to make Kegel exercises more challenging. These props can provide additional resistance, helping you build more strength.

It's crucial to remember that as you progress to intermediate Kegel exercises, the correct form is still paramount. Focus on contracting and relaxing the pelvic floor muscles properly, and avoid engaging other muscle groups, such as the buttocks or thighs. Additionally, be mindful of your breath, and do not hold your breath during exercises.

Before advancing to intermediate exercises, consult with a healthcare professional or physical therapist to ensure that you have a solid foundation and proper technique. They can provide personalized guidance, monitor your progress, and help you choose the most suitable exercises for your specific pelvic health goals. Over time, you can customize your Kegel routine to match your progress and maintain a strong, healthy pelvic floor.

5.2 Advanced Kegel Exercises

Once you have mastered basic and intermediate Kegel exercises and your pelvic floor muscles have become stronger and more coordinated, you can consider advanced Kegel exercises. These exercises are designed to further challenge and enhance the strength and endurance of your pelvic floor muscles. Here are some advanced Kegel exercises to explore:

1. **Kegel Progression: Pyramid Holds:** In this exercise, you'll gradually increase the duration of your pelvic floor muscle

contractions in a pyramid-like fashion. Start with a 5-second hold, then increase to 10 seconds, 15 seconds, and finally 20 seconds. After the 20-second hold, reverse the pyramid, working your way back down to 5 seconds. This exercise builds endurance.

2. **Kegel Balls or Weights:** Use Kegel balls or weights, which are specifically designed to provide resistance during Kegel exercises. Insert a Kegel ball or weight into your vagina, and then contract your pelvic floor muscles to hold it in place. Over time, you can gradually increase the weight of the ball or weight to challenge your muscles further.

3. **Kegel Squats:** Perform Kegel exercises while doing squats. Start with your feet shoulder-width apart and slowly lower your body into a squat position. Contract your pelvic floor muscles during the descent and release them as you return to the standing position. This exercise combines lower body strength training with pelvic floor engagement.

4. **Kegel Lunges:** Similar to Kegel squats, incorporate Kegel exercises into lunges. Take a step forward into a lunge, contracting your pelvic floor muscles as you lower your body. Release the contraction as you return to the starting position.

5. **Kegel Planks:** While holding a plank position (forearms and toes on the ground, body straight), contract your pelvic floor muscles. This exercise strengthens your core and pelvic floor simultaneously.

6. **Kegel Resistance Bands:** Attach resistance bands to your ankles and perform leg lifts while contracting your pelvic floor muscles. The resistance bands add challenge to your exercises, working both the pelvic floor and leg muscles.

7. **Kegel Yoga Poses:** Incorporate Kegel exercises into yoga poses that engage the pelvic floor, such as boat pose, bridge pose, and happy baby pose. This combines the benefits of yoga with Kegel exercises.

8. **Interval Contractions:**
   Alternate between short, quick contractions and longer, sustained contractions. For example, perform a series of 10 quick contractions, followed by a 30-second sustained contraction. Repeat this interval pattern.

When attempting advanced Kegel exercises, remember to maintain proper form and technique. Focus on contracting and relaxing the pelvic floor muscles correctly, and avoid overusing other muscle groups. It's also essential to be patient and progress at a pace that's comfortable for you. If you encounter any pain or discomfort, discontinue the exercise and consult with a healthcare professional or physical therapist for guidance.

Advanced Kegel exercises can provide significant benefits for pelvic health, sexual function, and overall well-being. However, they are not suitable for everyone, so it's advisable to seek professional guidance to ensure you're performing them safely and effectively.

5.3 Tracking Your Progress

Tracking your progress in your Kegel exercise routine is essential for maintaining motivation and ensuring you're moving toward your pelvic health goals. Here are some ways to monitor and measure your progress:

1. **Keep a Kegel Exercise Journal:** Create a dedicated journal or use a note-taking app

to record your daily or weekly Kegel exercise sessions. Include details such as the number of repetitions, the duration of contractions and relaxations, and any challenges or improvements you've experienced.

2. **Use a Kegel Exercise App:** There are numerous apps available that can help you track your Kegel exercises. These apps often provide guided routines, reminders, and progress tracking features. They can be a convenient way to monitor your daily exercises.

3. **Set Specific Goals:** Establish clear, achievable goals for your Kegel exercises. These goals might include improving urinary continence, enhancing

sexual satisfaction, or addressing specific pelvic health concerns. Setting targets will give you a sense of purpose and direction in your exercises.

4. **Measure Strength and Endurance:** Periodically assess your pelvic floor strength and endurance. This can be done by working with a physical therapist or using specialized devices designed to measure pelvic floor muscle strength.

5. **Check for Symptom Improvement:** If you began Kegel exercises to address specific symptoms, such as urinary incontinence or pelvic organ prolapse, assess whether these symptoms have improved over time. Reduced frequency

and severity of symptoms are positive indicators of progress.

6. **Photographic or Video Recordings:** With guidance from a healthcare professional, you may consider using photographic or video recordings to monitor your form and technique. This can help ensure that you're engaging the correct muscles during exercises.

7. **Seek Professional Feedback:** Consult with a healthcare professional or physical therapist at regular intervals. They can provide feedback on your progress, assess your technique, and adjust your exercise routine as needed.

8. **Regular Self-Assessments:** Perform self-assessments by periodically asking yourself how you feel during daily activities. Are you experiencing fewer incidents of incontinence? Is your sexual function improving? Are you feeling more in control of your pelvic health?

9. **Adjust Your Routine:** As you make progress, adapt your Kegel exercise routine. This might involve increasing the number of repetitions, holding contractions for longer periods, or adding more challenging exercises to your routine.

10. **Celebrate Achievements:** Acknowledge and celebrate your achievements and milestones. Recognizing your

progress can be a powerful motivator to continue with your Kegel exercises.

progress with Kegel exercises may be gradual, and the pace of improvement can vary from person to person. Be patient with yourself and understand that consistent effort is key to achieving your pelvic health goals. If you ever encounter difficulties or have concerns about your progress, don't hesitate to consult with a healthcare professional or physical therapist who can provide personalized guidance and support.

CHAPTER 6

Common Questions and Concerns

6.1 Can You Overdo Kegel Exercises?

While Kegel exercises offer numerous benefits for pelvic health and overall well-being, it is indeed possible to overdo them. Overexertion can lead to several issues, including muscle fatigue, discomfort, and counterproductive results. Here are some key considerations to avoid overdoing Kegel exercises:

1. **Muscle Fatigue:** Like any muscle group, the pelvic floor muscles can become fatigued

with excessive use. Overexertion can lead to muscle exhaustion and weaken the muscles rather than strengthening them.

2. **Ineffective Contractions:** Overdoing Kegel exercises can result in uncoordinated or ineffective contractions, where the muscles may not fully relax between contractions. Proper relaxation is essential for the overall health and function of these muscles.

3. **Discomfort or Pain:** Excessive contractions can cause discomfort, pain, or a feeling of pelvic pressure. If you experience pain during or after Kegel exercises, it's a sign that you may be overdoing them.

4. **Worsening Symptoms:** If you have specific pelvic health issues, such as pelvic pain, overdoing Kegel exercises can potentially exacerbate your symptoms. For some individuals, these exercises may not be appropriate or could even worsen existing conditions.

To avoid overdoing Kegel exercises:

- **Follow a Balanced Routine:** Stick to a well-balanced routine that includes the appropriate number of repetitions and sets. Over time, you can gradually increase the intensity and duration of your exercises.

- **Allow for Adequate Rest:** Ensure that you allow your pelvic floor muscles to fully relax between contractions. Proper relaxation is essential for muscle recovery and overall health.

- **Listen to Your Body:** Pay attention to how your body responds to the exercises. If you experience discomfort, pain, or fatigue, adjust your routine accordingly. It's essential to strike a balance between challenging your muscles and preventing overexertion.

- **Consult with a Professional:** If you're unsure about the appropriate number of repetitions, sets, or exercise intensity, or if you have specific pelvic health concerns, consult with a healthcare professional or physical therapist. They can provide personalized guidance tailored to your needs and goals.

- **Avoid Unnecessary Exercises:** Avoid doing Kegel exercises when they are not needed. For example, if you already have strong pelvic floor muscles, overtraining them can lead to issues. It's important to customize your exercise routine to your individual situation.

while Kegel exercises are highly beneficial for pelvic health, they should be approached with moderation and consideration of your unique circumstances. Consulting with a healthcare professional or physical therapist is an excellent way to ensure that you are performing Kegel exercises at the right level and intensity to meet your specific goals while avoiding overexertion.

6.2 Troubleshooting Common Issues

Kegel exercises, like any form of physical activity, can sometimes come with challenges and issues. Here are some common problems that people encounter with Kegel exercises and how to troubleshoot them:

Issue 1: Difficulty Identifying the Right Muscles

- **Troubleshooting:** If you have trouble finding the correct pelvic floor muscles, consider using the "stop the flow" method or the "finger test" to pinpoint them. You can also consult a healthcare professional or a physical therapist for guidance and assessment.

Issue 2: Lack of Progress

- **Troubleshooting:** If you feel that you're not making progress, ensure that you are doing the exercises consistently and correctly. If you're following a routine with adequate repetitions and sets and still not seeing improvement, consult a healthcare professional to assess your technique and provide personalized advice.

Issue 3: Overexertion

- **Troubleshooting:** If you experience discomfort, muscle fatigue, or pain, it's a sign of overexertion. Reduce the intensity of your exercises, ensure you're allowing for adequate relaxation between contractions, and consider consulting a healthcare professional for guidance on appropriate exercise levels.

Issue 4: Lack of Motivation

- **Troubleshooting:** Maintaining motivation for Kegel exercises can be a challenge. Create specific goals, use reminders, track your progress, and celebrate achievements to stay motivated. Joining support groups or forums with others who are also doing Kegel exercises can provide additional motivation.

Issue 5: Forgetfulness

- **Troubleshooting:** If you often forget to do your exercises, set reminders on your phone or use a Kegel exercise app to keep you on track. Incorporate Kegel exercises into your daily routine, such as during daily activities, to make them a natural part of your day.

Issue 6: Not Feeling Results

- **Troubleshooting:** If you don't notice any changes or improvements in your symptoms or pelvic health, consult with a healthcare professional to assess your specific situation. They can help identify the underlying causes and provide personalized guidance on how to tailor your exercises for better results.

Issue 7: Inconsistent Routine

- **Troubleshooting:** Staying consistent with Kegel exercises can be a challenge. Try to set a schedule, use reminders, and consider finding a workout partner or support group to keep you accountable.

Issue 8: Lack of Time

- **Troubleshooting:** If time is a barrier, remember that Kegel exercises can be done discreetly and take only a few minutes. You can incorporate them into your daily activities, such as during your commute or while watching TV, to make the most of your available time.

Issue 9: Apprehension About Technique

- **Troubleshooting:** If you're concerned about your technique, seek professional guidance. Consult with a healthcare professional or physical therapist who can assess your technique and provide instructions on how to perform Kegel exercises correctly.

Issue 10: Physical Discomfort

- **Troubleshooting:** If you experience physical discomfort or pain during or after Kegel exercises, stop the exercises immediately. Consult with a healthcare professional to rule out any underlying medical issues and get guidance on the appropriate exercise routine for your situation.

Troubleshooting common issues with Kegel exercises often involves a combination of adjusting your technique, maintaining consistency, setting goals, and seeking professional guidance when necessary. Personalizing your approach to Kegel exercises can help you overcome challenges and make the most of these exercises for your pelvic health and well-being.

6.3 Seeking Professional Guidance

Seeking professional guidance for your Kegel exercises can be highly beneficial, especially if you have specific pelvic health concerns, are experiencing challenges, or want to ensure that yo u are performing the exercises correctly. Here's how and when to seek professional guidance:

1. **Consult a Healthcare Professional:** If you are new to Kegel exercises or have specific pelvic health concerns, consider consulting a healthcare professional. A urologist, gynecologist, or physical therapist with expertise in pelvic health can assess your situation, provide personalized guidance, and recommend an appropriate exercise routine.

2. **Diagnose Pelvic Health Issues:** If you are experiencing symptoms like urinary incontinence, pelvic pain, or pelvic organ prolapse, a healthcare professional can help diagnose the underlying causes.

Identifying the root issues is crucial for tailoring your Kegel exercises to your needs.

3. **Assess Technique:** If you're unsure about your technique, a healthcare professional can assess your form and provide feedback to ensure that you are correctly engaging the pelvic floor muscles during your exercises.

4. **Customize Your Routine:** A professional can customize a Kegel exercise routine that aligns with your goals, whether that's improving continence, enhancing sexual function, or addressing specific pelvic health concerns.

5. **Progress Monitoring:** Regular check-ins with a healthcare

professional can help you monitor your progress and make necessary adjustments to your exercise routine as you advance.

6. **Treatment Plans:** In some cases, a healthcare professional may recommend additional treatments or interventions, such as biofeedback therapy, electrical stimulation, or other therapies, in conjunction with Kegel exercises to address specific pelvic health issues.

7. **Addressing Pelvic Pain:** If you experience pelvic pain or discomfort during or after Kegel exercises, consult a healthcare professional. Pelvic pain can have various causes, and a professional can help you determine the most appropriate

treatment or exercise modifications.

8. **Appropriate for Your Situation:** Kegel exercises are not suitable for everyone, and in some cases, they can worsen symptoms or create complications. Seeking professional guidance is essential to ensure that Kegel exercises are appropriate for your specific situation.

It's important to remember that professional guidance can provide you with the assurance that you are pursuing the right approach to Kegel exercises for your individual needs and goals. These exercises can be a valuable part of pelvic health, but they are most effective when tailored to your situation and performed correctly. Therefore, don't hesitate to reach out to a healthcare professional or physical therapist who specializes in pelvic health to get the guidance and support you require.

CHAPTER 7

Incorporating Kegels into Daily Life

7.1 Kegels for Men

Kegel exercises are often associated with women's health, but they are equally beneficial for men. They can help improve urinary and sexual health, promote better prostate health, and enhance overall pelvic floor strength. Here's how men can incorporate Kegel exercises into their daily lives:

1. Identify the Right Muscles:

- To start, identify your pelvic floor muscles. You can do this by trying to stop the flow of urine midstream. However, do not make a habit of this, as repeatedly stopping the flow of urine can lead to bladder issues. Visualize the muscles you use to prevent gas from passing, as these are the same muscles.

- Another method is to insert a clean finger into your rectum and contract the muscles. When you do this correctly, you should feel a gentle squeeze around your finger.

2. Perform Kegel Exercises:

- Once you've identified the right muscles, you can start incorporating Kegel exercises into your daily routine. These exercises involve contracting and relaxing the pelvic floor muscles.

- Start with the basic Kegel exercises as outlined earlier. These typically involve 3-10 second contractions followed by relaxation.

3. Create a Routine:

- Establish a routine for your Kegel exercises. Determine when and where you will do them, and stick to your schedule. Consistency is key to experiencing the benefits.

4. Integrate Kegels into Daily Activities:

- You can do Kegel exercises discreetly during daily activities such as sitting, standing, or walking. Focus on contracting and relaxing the pelvic floor muscles while you perform other tasks.

5. Use Reminders:

- Set reminders on your phone or use a Kegel exercise app to help you remember to do your exercises.

6. Combine Kegels with Other Activities:

- You can incorporate Kegel exercises into your fitness routine. For example, do Kegel exercises while lifting weights, or practice them during yoga, pilates, or core workouts.

7. Incorporate Kegels into Sexual Activity:

- Kegel exercises can enhance sexual function in men. Try practicing Kegels during sexual activity to improve control and pleasure.

8. Be Patient and Consistent:

- Results from Kegel exercises may take time to become noticeable. Be patient and consistent with your routine. Over time, you can adjust your exercises to make them more challenging and tailor them to your specific goals.

9. Seek Professional Guidance:

- If you have specific concerns or pelvic health issues, consider consulting a healthcare professional or physical therapist who specializes in men's pelvic health. They can provide personalized guidance and monitor your progress.

Kegel exercises are a valuable tool for men to enhance pelvic health, manage urinary incontinence, and improve sexual function. By incorporating them into your daily life, you can experience the full range of benefits these exercises offer.

7.2 Kegels for Women

Kegel exercises offer numerous benefits for women, such as improved pelvic health, urinary continence, and enhanced sexual function. Here's how women can incorporate Kegel exercises into their daily lives:

1. Identify the Right Muscles:

- To start, identify your pelvic floor muscles. You can do this by trying to stop the flow of urine midstream. However, it's essential not to make a habit of this, as frequently stopping the flow of urine can lead to bladder issues. Visualize the muscles you use to prevent gas from passing, as these are the same muscles.

- Another method is to insert a clean finger into your vagina and contract the muscles. When you do this correctly, you should feel a gentle squeeze around your finger.

2. Perform Kegel Exercises:

- Once you've identified the right muscles, you can start incorporating Kegel exercises into your daily routine. These exercises involve contracting and relaxing the pelvic floor muscles.

- Begin with the basic Kegel exercises as outlined earlier. These typically involve 3-10 second contractions followed by relaxation.

3. Create a Routine:

- Establish a routine for your Kegel exercises. Determine when and where you will do them, and stick to your schedule. Consistency is key to experiencing the benefits.

4. Integrate Kegels into Daily Activities:

- You can do Kegel exercises discreetly during daily activities such as sitting, standing, or walking. Focus on contracting and relaxing the pelvic floor muscles while you perform other tasks.

5. Use Reminders:

- Set reminders on your phone or use a Kegel exercise app to help you remember to do your exercises.

6. Combine Kegels with Other Activities:

- You can incorporate Kegel exercises into your fitness routine. For example, do Kegel exercises while doing yoga, pilates, or core workouts.

7. Incorporate Kegels into Sexual Activity:

- Kegel exercises can enhance sexual function in women. Try practicing Kegels during sexual activity to improve control and pleasure.

8. Be Patient and Consistent:

- Results from Kegel exercises may take time to become noticeable. Be patient and consistent with your routine. Over time, you can adjust your exercises to make them more challenging and tailor them to your specific goals.

9. Seek Professional Guidance:

- If you have specific concerns or pelvic health issues, consider consulting a healthcare professional or physical therapist who specializes in women's pelvic health. They can provide personalized guidance and monitor your progress.

7.3 Maintaining a Healthy Pelvic Floor

A healthy pelvic floor is essential for overall well-being, and it's crucial to maintain its health throughout life. Here are some tips to help both men and women maintain a healthy pelvic floor:

1. Stay Hydrated:

- Proper hydration supports urinary health and helps prevent urinary tract infections. Drink an adequate amount of water daily to keep your urinary system functioning optimally.

2. Maintain a Healthy Diet:

- A balanced diet that includes plenty of fiber can help prevent constipation. Constipation can strain the pelvic floor muscles and lead to pelvic floor issues. Incorporate fruits, vegetables, and whole grains into your meals.

3. Manage Body Weight:

- Maintaining a healthy body weight can reduce pressure on the pelvic floor. Excess weight can strain the pelvic muscles and lead to incontinence or pelvic organ prolapse.

4. Engage in Regular Exercise:

- Regular physical activity can help maintain overall health, including pelvic health. Activities such as walking, swimming, and yoga can be beneficial. Additionally, specific pelvic floor exercises, like Kegels, can be included in your exercise routine.

5. Avoid Smoking:

- Smoking can contribute to chronic coughing, which can strain the pelvic floor muscles. Quitting smoking can improve your overall health and help prevent such strains.

6. Proper Lifting Techniques:

- When lifting heavy objects, use your legs, not your back, to avoid putting excessive pressure on the pelvic floor. Engage your core and use proper lifting techniques to protect these muscles.

7. Support Your Pelvic Floor During Pregnancy:

- If you're pregnant, work with a healthcare provider or physical therapist who specializes in women's health to develop a plan for maintaining your pelvic floor during and after pregnancy.

8. Don't Delay Urination:

- Urinate when you feel the urge to avoid overfilling your bladder. Delaying urination can put pressure on the pelvic floor muscles and lead to urinary issues.

9. Practice Proper Posture:

- Maintain good posture to support the alignment of the pelvis and pelvic floor. Use ergonomically designed chairs if you have a sedentary job.

10. Manage Chronic Health Conditions:

- Certain chronic health conditions, like diabetes and high blood pressure, can affect pelvic health. Managing these conditions with medical guidance can help protect your pelvic floor.

11. Pelvic Floor Physical Therapy:

- Consider pelvic floor physical therapy if you have specific concerns or issues related to your pelvic floor. A specialized physical therapist can assess your condition and provide tailored exercises and treatment.

12. Regular Health Check-ups:

- Regular check-ups with your healthcare provider can help identify and address pelvic health issues early, before they become more challenging to treat.

13. Maintain Sexual Health:

- A satisfying sex life can help promote overall pelvic health. Maintain open communication with your partner and address any concerns you may have related to sexual function.

14. Emotional Well-being:

- Emotional well-being is closely tied to physical health. Managing stress and anxiety can help reduce muscle tension and promote pelvic health.

15. Consult a Specialist:

- If you have specific concerns or experience symptoms related to your pelvic floor, consult a healthcare specialist, such as a urologist, gynecologist, or physical therapist who specializes in pelvic health.

Maintaining a healthy pelvic floor is an ongoing process that involves lifestyle choices, regular exercise, and seeking professional guidance when needed. Prioritizing pelvic health can contribute to overall well-being and quality of life.

Made in the USA
Coppell, TX
16 March 2024